300 Questions and Answers in Surgical Nursing and Anaesthesia

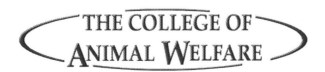

THE COLLEGE OF ANIMAL WELFARE

300 Questions and Answers in Surgical Nursing and Anaesthesia

The College of Animal Welfare

3/06

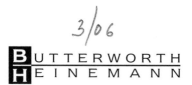

EDINBURGH LONDON NEW YORK OXFORD PHILADELPHIA
ST LOUIS SYDNEY TORONTO 2000

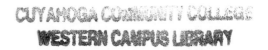

Butterworth-Heinemann Ltd
An imprint of Elsevier Limited
Robert Stevenson House,
1-3 Baxter's Place,
Leith Walk,
Edinburgh EH1 3AF

First published 2000
Reprinted 2002, 2004

British Library Cataloguing in Publication Data

ISBN 0 7506 4698 5

your source for books,
journals and multimedia
in the health sciences
www.elsevierhealth.com

Typeset by Keyword Typesetting Services, Wallington
Printed and bound in Great Britain by MPG Books Ltd, Bodmin, Cornwall

Contents

Acknowledgements

The College is most grateful for the help of the following colleagues in the preparation of this book:

C. Allan
B. Cooper
W. Fulcher
D. Gould
A. Jeffrey
H. Orpet
A. Thomas

Introduction

How the book is organized

This book of surgical nursing and anaesthesia questions has been produced in response to further requests for more multiple choice questions. It contains 300 questions covering surgical nursing and anaesthesia. After the questions is a list of correct answers.

How to use the book

Do your revision first, then select a range of question numbers at random. Do this without looking at the questions in advance. You should be able to complete and finish one multiple choice question per minute, allowing time for a thorough read of the question and the options before selecting the correct answer.

Questions

1) *A gastropexy might be indicated in the management of which condition?*

   a) Gastric foreign body
   b) Gastric neoplasm
   c) Gastric torsion
   d) Haemorrhagic gastro-enteritis

2) *The condition which could be an indication for performing a urethrostomy in a male animal is:*

   a) a ruptured bladder
   b) hydronephrosis
   c) urethral calculi
   d) ectopic ureter

3) *Animals with lymphosarcoma are MOST commonly treated using which type of tumour therapy?*

   a) Chemotherapy
   b) Radiotherapy
   c) Surgery
   d) Isotopes

4) *Cataracts affect which part of the eye?*

   a) Lens
   b) Cornea
   c) Aqueous humour
   d) Retina

5) *Which ONE of the following tumours that affect bone is benign?*

   a) Osteosarcoma
   b) Chondrosarcoma
   c) Osteochondroma
   d) Fibrosarcoma

6) *A drain could be used in which ONE of the following situations?*

   a) A shallow wound healing by second intention
   b) A cystotomy
   c) A deep wound where tissue has been removed leaving dead space
   d) A small surgical wound healing by first intention

7) *A Penrose drain with gauze down the central lumen of the drain is called a:*

   a) Penrose drain
   b) cigarette drain
   c) sump-Penrose
   d) tube drain

8) *Which ONE of the following is NOT a method by which a passive drain works?*

   a) Gravitation
   b) Overflow
   c) Capillary action
   d) Suction

9) *When should a Heimlich valve be used?*

   a) In cases of pleural effusion and pneumothorax
   b) In cases of pneumothorax only
   c) In cases where only fluid is being drained
   d) When draining the abdomen

10) *Which ONE of the following surgical procedures could be performed at the same time as a dental scale and polish?*

   a) Bitch spay
   b) Fracture repair
   c) Small wart removal
   d) None of the above

11) *Which ONE of the following is a congenital disease of the oral cavity?*

    a) Cleft palate
    b) Gum epulides
    c) Gingivitis
    d) Sialagogitis

12) *Which ONE of the following is NOT a symptom of megaoesophagus?*

    a) Weight loss
    b) Aspiration pneumonia
    c) Regurgitation
    d) Vomiting

13) *Intussusception is linked with which ONE of the following:*

    a) diarrhoea
    b) constipation
    c) a heavy burden of endoparasites
    d) all of the above

14) *Rectal tumours can be visualized via:*

    a) cystoscopy
    b) proctoscopy
    c) colonoscopy
    d) rectoscopy

15) *Skin fold dermatitis is MOST likely to occur in which ONE of the following breeds*

   a) Labrador
   b) Saluki
   c) Sharpei
   d) Collie

16) *A breed COMMONLY associated with anal furunculosis is:*

   a) Old English Bull Terrier
   b) Sharpei
   c) German Shepherd Dog
   d) Cocker Spaniel

17) *What other procedure SHOULD be carried out when an anal adenoma is removed from an elderly male dog?*

   a) A chat to his owners about diet
   b) Castration
   c) Anal sac removal
   d) Prostatectomy

18) *Which ONE of the following analgesics is useful for laryngeal surgery because of its antitussive qualities?*

   a) Burtorphanol
   b) Bupivicaine
   c) Buprenorphine
   d) Butyrophenone

19) *Which ONE of the following is NOT associated with brachycephalic airway obstruction syndrome?*

   a) Narrow nares
   b) Overlong soft palate
   c) Narrow trachea
   d) Hypoplastic bronchi

20) *The term used to describe the procedure of forcing sterile saline through a urinary catheter to dislodge urethral calculi is:*

   a) hydropulsion
   b) retropulsion
   c) urethropulsion
   d) hyperpulsion

21) *The disease of the ear that OFTEN affects the organ of balance is:*

   a) otitis externa
   b) otitis interna
   c) otitis media
   d) aural haematoma

22) *Which ONE of the following pieces of equipment gives the BEST assurance that sterilisation has taken place?*

   a) Bowie-Dick tape
   b) TST strips
   c) Browne's tubes
   d) Autoclave tape

23) *The normal incision for an emergency tracheotomy is caudal to:*

   a) the first or second pair of tracheal rings
   b) the second or third pair of tracheal rings
   c) the fourth or fifth pair of tracheal rings
   d) any tracheal rings

24) *Which ONE of the following is NOT a common sign of shock?*

   a) Pale mucous membranes
   b) Capillary refill time of 1–2 seconds
   c) Cold extremities
   d) Collapse

25) *Which ONE of the following is the MOST common type of shock?*

   a) Neurogenic shock
   b) Psychogenic shock
   c) Cardiogenic shock
   d) Hypovolaemic shock

26) *An example of an incomplete fracture is a:*

   a) comminuted fracture
   b) transverse fracture
   c) fissured fracture
   d) compound fracture

27) *Another name for a fracture through a grown plate is a:*

   a) Salter–Harris fracture
   b) Condylar fracture
   c) Diaphyseal fracture
   d) Epiphyseal fracture

28) *What is the term given to the union of a fracture that is healed in a deformed position?*

   a) Non-union
   b) Nil union
   c) Malunion
   d) Any of the above

29) *Fracture disease occurs MORE COMMONLY with which type of fracture fixation:*

   a) external coaptation
   b) ASIF
   c) Venables plates and screws
   d) Kirschner–Ehmer fixator

30) *How long does plaster of paris take to reach its full strength?*

   a) 12 hours
   b) 24 hours
   c) 36 hours
   d) 48 hours

31) *A common type of extension splint is the:*

   a) Kirschner–Ehmer splint
   b) Kirschner–Schroeder splint
   c) Schroeder–Thomas splint
   d) Thomas–Ehmer splint

32) *Name the plate pictured below:*

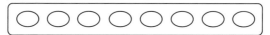

   a) Sherman plate
   b) ASIF. plate
   c) Burns plate
   d) Venables plate

33) *Name the plate pictured below:*

   a) Sherman plate
   b) ASIF. plate
   c) Burns plate
   d) Venables plate

34) *Which ONE of the following is NOT a feature of a Rush pin?*

   a) It is curved
   b) The top of the pin is bent over to form a hook
   c) It is often used to anchor ephiphyseal fragments back onto the shaft of the bone
   d) It is always used singly

35) *Which ONE of the following bandages would you put on a dislocated hip that has just undergone closed reduction?*

a) Thomas sling
b) Velpeau sling
c) Ehmer sling
d) Kirschner sling

36) *A wound that is caused by a scalpel is MOST likely to heal via:*

a) granulation
b) first intention healing
c) second intention healing
d) skin graft

37) *A fresh traumatic wound (less than six hours old) can be classed as a:*

a) clean wound
b) clean–contaminated wound
c) contaminated wound
d) dirty (infected) wound

38) *A surgical wound, made under aseptic conditions, becomes which type of wound if the surgeon punctures his or her glove while operating?*

a) A clean wound
b) A clean–contaminated wound
c) A contaminated wound
d) A dirty (infected) wound

39) *Which ONE of the following types of assisted feeding is considered the BEST for cases needing feeding for longer than seven days?*

   a) Percutaneous endoscopic gastrotomy tube
   b) Naso-oesophageal tube
   c) Naso-gastric tube
   d) Pharyngostomy tube

40) *The name given to an abnormal tract that connects two epithelial surfaces is:*

   a) cellulitus
   b) a sinus
   c) a fistula
   d) an abscess

41) *The animal MOST likely to suffer from hypothermia during surgery is:*

   a) a mouse
   b) a guinea pig
   c) a cat
   d) a dog

42) *An adenocarcinoma is:*

   a) a benign tumour of fibrous tissue
   b) a malignant tumour of fibrous tissue
   c) a benign tumour of glandular tissue
   d) a malignant tumour of glandular tissue

43) *The CORRECT term for a permanent opening into the trachea is:*

   a) tracheotomy
   b) tracheostomy
   c) trachectomy
   d) tracheapexy

44) *For which ONE of the following reasons may a veterinary surgeon MOST COMMONLY perform a cystotomy?*

   a) To dissect out a portion of the bladder wall when a tumour is present
   b) To remove bladder stones
   c) To unblock the urethra when urinary calculi are causing a blockage
   d) None of the above

45) *A film covering the teeth, made up of bacteria, food particles and saliva, is known as:*

   a) dental calculus
   b) gingivitis
   c) plaque
   d) tartar

46) *The correct suffix for a term describing the surgical removal of a structure is:*

a) -ectomy
b) -itis
c) -ostomy
d) -otomy

47) *The scaling of teeth should NOT be performed at the same time as other major surgery because:*

a) different antibiotics may be required for the two different procedures
b) scaling increases the time the animal is under general anaesthetic, and therefore increases the anaesthetic risk
c) scaling can produce oral discomfort for some days afterwards, so the patient is less willing to eat and takes longer to recover from surgery
d) scaling releases bacteria from the mouth into the blood stream, leading to an increased risk of wound infection

48) *What is the name of the technique whereby a needle is put through the abdominal wall in order to drain urine from the bladder?*

a) Abdominocentesis
b) Cystocentesis
c) Percutaneous compression
d) Thoracocentesis

49) *Which ONE of the following is NOT a causative factor in dental disease?*

    a) Caries
    b) Distemper
    c) Halitosis
    d) Pulpitis

50) *What is the MOST urgent procedure in gastric dilatation/volvulus syndrome?*

    a) Intravenous fluid
    b) Decompression of the stomach
    c) Passing an endotracheal tube
    d) Returning the stomach to its normal position

51) *Collapsing trachea is MOST commonly seen in:*

    a) German Shepherd Dogs
    b) Labrador Retrievers
    c) Corgis
    d) Yorkshire Terriers

52) *Hysterotomy describes:*

    a) removal of the uterus
    b) removal of the ovaries and the uterus
    c) temporary opening into the uterus
    d) none of the above

53) *The BEST preventative treatment of vaginal hyperplasia is:*

   a) ovariohysterectomy
   b) surgical resection
   c) progestogen therapy
   d) nothing, because it only occurs in immature bitches that will eventually grow out of it

54) *Which ONE of the following would NOT be a reason for castration?*

   a) To reduce excessive libido
   b) To reduce roaming
   c) To increase unwanted breeding
   d) To prevent roaming

55) *Pus within the anterior chamber in the eye is known as:*

   a) entropion
   b) ureitis
   c) proptosis
   d) hypopion

56) *What device would you use to examine the rectum?*

   a) An auroscope
   b) A proctoscope
   c) A laryngoscope
   d) An opthalmoscope

57) *Cryosurgery, used in the treatment of tissue, is by application of:*

   a) heat
   b) cytotoxic drugs
   c) extreme cold
   d) radiation

58) *Trauma to the central nervous system may result in which type of shock?*

   a) vasculogenic
   b) neurogenic
   c) endotoxic
   d) cardiogenic

59) *An overdose of acepromazine is LIKELY to cause:*

   a) neurogenic shock
   b) vasculogenic shock
   c) cardiogenic shock
   d) endotoxic shock

60) *What hormone is responsible for retaining sodium?*

   a) Antidiuretic hormone (ADH}
   b) Aldosterone
   c) Adrenaline
   d) None of the above

61) *Which ONE of the following is NOT usually a causative factor in hypothermia?*

   a) Exposure to cold
   b) Malnutrition
   c) Inactivity
   d) The use of rebreathing circuits

62) *Which ONE of the following signs is NOT usually indicative of hypothermia?*

   a) shivering
   b) pale mucous membranes
   c) increased pulse rate
   d) lethargy

63) *Which ONE of the following precautions is the LEAST used in the prevention of hypothermia during a surgical procedure?*

   a) Placing the animal on a heat pad throughout the procedure
   b) Giving warmed fluids subcutaneously
   c) Careful patient preparation, ensuring the animal does not get too wet
   d) Ensuring the environmental temperature in the theatre is relatively high

64) *To prevent hyperthermia, additional heat sources
     should be removed once core temperature has been
     reached at:*

   a) 38.0°C
   b) 38.5°C
   c) 39.0°C
   d) 39.5°C

65) *Which ONE of the following is NOT usually indicative
     of hyperthermia?*

   a) Decreased pulse rate
   b) Shock
   c) Cyanosis
   d) Increased salivation

66) *The MOST important first aid treatment of
     hyperthermia is to:*

   a) cool the patient
   b) ensure a patent airway
   c) put in a cool cage and check core temperature
      every fifteen minutes
   d) give cool intravenous fluids

67) *Dehiscence is defined as:*

a) poor blood supply to a wound caused by bruizing of the surrounding tissues
b) skin necrosis caused by excessively tight sutures
c) the formation of a seromia on the site of the surgical wound
d) wound breakdown

68) *Which ONE of the following dressings is NOT indicated to encourage sloughing of necrotic tissue in a large wound?*

a) A dry non-adherent dressing
b) An alginate dressing
c) An occlusive hydrocolloid dressing
d) Successive wet packs made up with sterile saline

69) *In the process of wound healing, organisation is defined as:*

a) the process by which inflammatory tissue is removed once an abscess is drained
b) the replacement of damaged tissue by scar tissue
c) the replacement of destroyed tissue by similar functional tissue
d) the return of the tissue to the state it was in before the start of the inflammatory process

70) *A skin graft of small plugs of dermis implanted in matching incisions in the granulation tissue is known as:*

   a) a mesh graft
   b) a pinch graft
   c) a stamp graft
   d) a strip graft

71) *Which ONE of the following is NOT a disadvantage in the use of drains in surgical wounds?*

   a) Drains may allow infection to gain access to the body
   b) The animal must be prevented from trying to remove the drain, often by wearing an Elizabethan collar
   c) The presence of a drain will usually increase the time taken for the original surgical wound to heal
   d) Drains act as foreign bodies within the tissues

72) *An inflammatory fluid containing dead tissue and leukocytes is called:*

   a) synovial fluid
   b) ulceration
   c) exudate
   d) pus

73) *A localized accumulation of dead and viable neutrophils in a cavity lined with fibrous tissue is called:*

   a) an abscess
   b) cellulitis
   c) a cyst
   d) an ulcer

74) *A sutured surgical wound in the oral mucosa is defined as:*

   a) a clean–contaminated wound
   b) a clean wound
   c) a contaminated wound
   d) an infected wound

75) *An allograft is a skin graft that:*

   a) has come from a different animal of the same species
   b) has come from an animal of a different species
   c) has come from elsewhere on the same animal
   d) includes only the epidermis and a small sliver of dermis

76) *An inflammatory reaction where pus is distributed through cleavage planes and tissue space is called:*

   a) a cold abscess
   b) an abscess
   c) cellulitis
   d) ulceration

77) *Which ONE of the following is NOT a cardinal sign of inflammation?*

   a) Normal limb movement
   b) Oedema
   c) Erythema
   d) Algesia

78) *Inflammation will NOT be caused by:*

   a) tumours
   b) burns
   c) bacterial spores
   d) viruses

79) *Pain associated with inflammation is due to:*

   a) pressure on nerve endings
   b) pressure on muscle fibres
   c) pressure on blood vessels
   d) pressure on bone ends

80) *Cell death associated with the loss of local blood supply and putrefaction of the tissues by bacteria is called:*

   a) necrosis
   b) gangrene
   c) abscessation
   d) degeneration

81) *Which ONE of the following drugs would NOT be indicated in the treatment of acute inflammation?*

   a) Paracetamol
   b) Aspirin
   c) Carprofen
   d) Phenylbutazone

82) *Treatment of ulcers does NOT include:*

   a) providing drainage
   b) removing the inciting cause
   c) treating any secondary bacterial infection
   d) providing temporary protection for the healing surface

83) *Examples of labile cells include:*

   a) cells of endocrine tissue
   b) cells of fibrous tissue
   c) cells of skeletal tissue
   d) cells of lymphoid tissue

84) *Examples of stable cells include:*

   a) cells of endocrine tissue
   b) cells of epithelial tissue
   c) blood cells
   d) cells of lymphoid tissue

85) *In a surgical list, which ONE should be the first case?*

   a) Lipoma removal
   b) Abscess debridement
   c) Ovariohysterectomy
   d) Excizion arturoplasty

86) *An operative wound made under aseptic conditions, penetrating the respiratory tract, is known as a:*

   a) clean wound
   b) clean–contaminated wound
   c) contaminated wound
   d) dirty (infected) wound

87) *Which ONE of the following is NOT a complication of wound healing?*

   a) Erythema
   b) Haematoma
   c) Odour
   d) Sterility

88) *From the list of procedures below, which ONE should be performed last?*

   a) Lipoma removal
   b) Abscess debridement
   c) Ovariohysterectomy
   d) Excizion arturoplasty

89) *A blind-ended tract, lined with granulation tissue and usually leading to an abscess cavity, is called a:*

a) hernia
b) abscess
c) fistula
d) sinus

90) *A seroma is MOST likely to occur after:*

a) bitch spay
b) mammary tumour removal
c) discectomy
d) femoral head arthroplasty

91) *Drains are NOT indicated for:*

a) abolishing dead space in wounds
b) drainage of contaminated wounds
c) full thickness skin grafts
d) removal of air from body cavities

92) *A fracture with an overlying open wound is classified as:*

a) avulsed
b) pathological
c) open
d) greenstick

93) *External coaptation is the term used to describe:*

   a) external/internal fixation
   b) intramedullary pinning
   c) plating
   d) casting materials

94) *Pain, swelling, heat, erythema and loss of normal function are signs of:*

   a) infection
   b) inflammation
   c) resolution
   d) necrosis

95) *What is resolution?*

   a) Replacement of damaged tissue by similar tissue
   b) Destruction of tissue
   c) Scar formation
   d) Return to normal with little or no damage

96) *What type of wound healing would you expect following a surgical incision?*

   a) Granulation
   b) Healing by second intention
   c) Healing by first intention
   d) Regeneration

97) *Which ONE of the following offers good residual efficacy after scrubbing up?*

    a) Cetavlon
    b) Hibiscrub
    c) Pevidine
    d) Savlon

98) *At what temperature does Bowie-Dick tape turn colour?*

    a) 131°C
    b) 151°C
    c) 121°C
    d) 112°C

99) *Which ONE of the following is a hydrocolloid dressing?*

    a) Melolin
    b) Primapore
    c) Allevyn
    d) Gauze swab

100) *What type of drain requires a suction pump?*

    a) Open
    b) Closed passive
    c) Closed active
    d) Penrose

101) *Which ONE of the following is NOT associated with the formation of pus?*

   a) Pyothorax
   b) Cellulitis
   c) Pyrosis
   d) Pyometra

102) *Which ONE of the following types of skin graft would involve transferring a section of skin to an adjacent area?*

   a) Pedicle graft
   b) Subdermal plexus skin flap
   c) Free skin graft
   d) Strip graft

103) *Which type of rupture or hernia can cause necrosis of tissues?*

   a) Incarcerated
   b) Strangulated
   c) Reducible
   d) Irreducible

104) *Which type of hernia is COMMONLY the result of direct trauma?*

   a) Umbilical
   b) Diaphragmatic
   c) Perineal
   d) Inguinal

105) *Which ONE of the following is a malignant tumour?*

   a) Lipoma
   b) Adenoma
   c) Fibrosarcoma
   d) Fibroma

106) *Which ONE of the following is a malignant tumour of bone?*

   a) Lymphosarcoma
   b) Adenocarcinoma
   c) Fibrocareinoma
   d) Oesteosarcoma

107) *What is a carcinogen?*

   a) A drug used to treat cancer
   b) An agent that causes normal cells to become malignant
   c) A malignant tumour of the epithelium
   d) A malignant tumour of the intestine

108) *Which ONE of the following is NOT a treatment for malignant tumours?*

   a) Cryosurgery
   b) Radiotherapy
   c) Chemosis
   d) Chemotherapy

109) *Which ONE of the following terms relates to a flaccid dilatation of the oesophagus?*

   a) Megaoesophagus
   b) Oesophagoscopy
   c) Oesophagitis
   d) Oesophagotomy

110) *Which ONE of the following terms means anchoring the stomach to the abdominal wall?*

   a) gastrotomy
   b) gastropexy
   c) gastropathy
   d) gastroplasty

111) *In a suspected case of gastric dilatation/volvulus, what would you advise the owner to do?*

   a) Monitor the animal and come to the surgery next day
   b) Bring the animal to the surgery straight away to have a stomach tube passed
   c) Exercise the animal to relieve the discomfort
   d) Make the animal vomit

112) *Which ONE of the following would NOT require an end to end anastomosis following surgical intervention?*

   a) Intussusception
   b) Removal of an intestinal carcinoma
   c) Enterectomy due to an intestinal foreign body
   d) Enterotomy

113) *Which ONE of the following conditions is NOT inherited?*

    a) Polydactyly
    b) Entropion
    c) Hip dysplasia
    d) Imperforate anus

114) *Cystocentesis is:*

    a) making an opening into the bladder
    b) the surgical excision of a cyst
    c) a sterile technique to empty the bladder or collect a urine sample
    d) the removal of bladder calculi

115) *Which ONE of the following is NOT a method of removing a urinary obstruction?*

    a) Cystotomy
    b) Urethrostomy
    c) Urethrotomy
    d) Cystocentesis

116) *Orchidectomy is:*

    a) removal of the prostrate gland
    b) removal of the testicles
    c) failure of the testicles to descend
    d) freeing a retained testicle and placing it in the scrotum

117) *Orchidectomy is NOT performed for which of the following conditions?*

   a) Testicular tumour
   b) Prostate disease
   c) Anal adenoma
   d) Perianal fistula

118) *Surgical removal of the ovaries and uterus is called:*

   a) hysterectomy
   b) hysterotomy
   c) ovariectomy
   d) ovariohysterectomy

119) *Elective hysterectomy should be performed:*

   a) during oestrus
   b) four weeks after the start of oestrus
   c) four weeks before the expected start of oestrus
   d) eight weeks after the end of oestrus

120) *Which is NOT a sign of pyometra?*

   a) Polydipsia
   b) Pyrexia
   c) Polyphagia
   d) Vaginal discharge

121) *A hysterotomy is performed for what reason?*

    a) An infected uterus
    b) Uveitis
    c) Dystocia
    d) Suspected neoplasm

122) *Laryngeal paralysis is often seen in:*

    a) underweight Labrador Retrievers
    b) overweight Labrador Retrievers
    c) underweight Yorkshire Terriers
    d) overweight Yorkshire Terriers

123) *A surgical opening into the nasal cavity is a:*

    a) rhinotomy
    b) rhinoscopy
    c) rhinorrhoea
    d) rhinopathy

124) *Which procedure would be carried out in an emergency to relieve an obstructed airway?*

    a) Tracheotomy
    b) Tracheostomy
    c) Thoracocentesis
    d) Thoracotomy

125) *The presence of blood in the pleural cavity is called:*

a) pneumothorax
b) haemoptysis
c) haemothorax
d) thoracocentesis

126) *Why are animals starved before general anaesthesia?*

a) To save the owners worry on the day of operation
b) Because gaseous anaesthetics are absorbed better through an empty stomach
c) To minimize the risk of vomiting during the procedure
d) None of the above

127) *For how long should items be aired after sterilization using the Anprolene sterilizer?*

a) 2 hours
b) 4 hours
c) 12 hours
d) 24 hours

128) *Which type of skin graft is made up of small squares of dermis implanted in the granulation bed?*

a) Pinch graft
b) Stamp graft
c) Strip graft
d) Mesh graft

129) *The correct suffix for a term describing the surgical removal of all or part of a structure is:*

   a) -ostomy
   b) -ectomy
   c) -itis
   d) -otomy

130) *A tracheotomy tube should be cleaned to remove any accumulated mucus:*

   a) daily
   b) two to three times daily
   c) every two to three hours
   d) every hour

131) *A papilloma is a:*

   a) benign, wart-like tumour of epithelial cells
   b) benign tumour of fibrous tissue
   c) benign tumour of epithelial melanocytes
   d) benign tumour of adipose tissue

132) *Which ONE of the following methods of sterilization should ideally NOT be used with cutting instruments?*

   a) Ethylene oxide
   b) Hot air oven
   c) Radiation
   d) Autoclave

133) *Cat gut comes from which animal?*

   a) Pig
   b) Sheep
   c) Cow
   d) Goat

134) *A to and fro circuit can be classed as which type of anaesthetic circuit?*

   a) Open
   b) Closed
   c) Semi-open
   d) Semi-closed

135) *Which ONE of the following metals is NOT used for surgical instruments?*

   a) Martensitic stainless steel
   b) Tungsten carbide
   c) Bromium-plated carbon steel
   d) Austenitic stainless steel

136) *Which ONE of the following should NOT be used in the cleaning of instruments?*

   a) cold water
   b) soap
   c) ultrasound cleaner
   d) detergent

137) *Which ONE of the following instruments is primarily used to hold organs and tissues, to allow exposure of the operating field?*

   a) Forceps
   b) Rongeurs
   c) Osteotome
   d) Retractor

138) *Which ONE of the following features does NOT classify surgical scissors?*

   a) The type of surgery they are used for
   b) The cutting edge of the blade
   c) The type of points they have
   d) The shape of the blade

139) *When performing cryosurgery how low must the temperature fall to achieve optimum lethal temperature?*

   a) −20°C
   b) −25°C
   c) −15°C
   d) −10°C

140) *Which ONE of the following is generally the refrigerant of choice for cryosurgery?*

   a) Liquid helium
   b) Liquid nitrogen
   c) Liquid hydrogen
   d) Liquid oxygen

141) *Which ONE of the following is NOT a requirement for storage after sterilization?*

a) Dust free conditions
b) Dry conditions
c) Darkened conditions
d) Well ventilated conditions

142) *Which ONE of the following CANNOT be used to sterilize an endoscope?*

a) Ethylene oxide
b) Hot air oven
c) Gluteraldehyde
d) Irradiation

143) *Which ONE of the following instruments has cupped jaws, and nibbles bones?*

a) Chisel
b) Curette
c) Rongeur
d) Osteotome

144) *Which ONE of the following is an example of an absorbable suture material?*

a) Polybutester
b) Polyamide
c) Polydioxanone
d) Polyethelene

145) *Which ONE of the following is an example of a non-absorbable suture material?*

    a) Polydioxanone

    b) Polypropylene

    c) Polyglactin 910

    d) Polyglycolic acid

146) *Which ONE of the following describes a needle with suture material attached?*

    a) Fixed

    b) Swaged

    c) Eyed

    d) Swaggered

147) *Which ONE of the following types of surgery is NOT elective?*

    a) Correction of a prolapsed eye

    b) Mastectomy of a benign tumour

    c) Ovariohysterectomy

    d) Dew claw removal

148) *Which surgical term describes the removal of necrotic tissue?*

    a) Exudate

    b) Incision

    c) Debridement

    d) Retraction

149) *Which ONE of the following does NOT have to be sterile during a surgical procedur?:*

   a) Drapes
   b) Gloves
   c) Mask
   d) Gown

150) *Which ONE of the following is NOT likely to cause dehiscence of an abdominal incision?*

   a) Vomiting
   b) Thick suture material
   c) Wound infection
   d) Stormy anaesthesia recovery

151) *The main goal of aseptic surgical technique is to prevent contamination of the:*

   a) operating personnel
   b) sterile field
   c) surgical wound
   d) surgical instruments

152) *Which personnel should face away from the sterile field during a surgical procedure?*

   a) All personnel
   b) Non-scrubbed personnel
   c) Scrubbed personnel
   d) None of the above

153) *What is the correct term for the removal of a kidney?*

    a) Nephrostomy
    b) Nephrectomy
    c) Nephrotomy
    d) Nephroscopy

154) *Which ONE of the following suture materials is badly damaged by steam steriliation:*

    a) polyglycolic acid
    b) nylon
    c) polypropylene
    d) silk

155) *Tissue forceps are best for grasping:*

    a) skin
    b) bone
    c) calculi
    d) fascia

156) *A nosocomial infection is one arizeng from the patient's:*

    a) blood stream
    b) environment
    c) respiratory system
    d) skin

157) *Which ONE of the following is a hand-held retractor?*

   a) Gossett
   b) West
   c) Langenbeck
   d) Balfour

158) *Which type of refractor is used for visualisation during abdominal surgery?*

   a) Gelpi
   b) Balfour
   c) Hohmann
   d) Travers

159) *Which ONE is NOT an example of a plate used for fracture fixation?*

   a) Venables
   b) West
   c) Sherman
   d) Dynamic compression

160) *When using ASIF technique, which drill bit size would be used for a 2.7 mm screw?*

   a) 2.0
   b) 2.7
   c) 3.2
   d) 1.5

161) *Which ONE of the following is NOT an example of internal fixation of a fracture?*

    a) Kuntscher nail
    b) Rush pins
    c) Tension band wiring
    d) Thomas splint

162) *ASIF plates are also known as:*

    a) Venables plates
    b) Sherman plates
    c) dynamic compression plates
    d) Burns plates

163) *Freedom from infection by the exclusion of micro-organisms and spores describes:*

    a) antisepsis
    b) sepsis
    c) asepsis
    d) disinfection

164) *Endogenous micro-organisms are those which:*

    a) are found on the skin
    b) come from within the patient's body
    c) are found on the coat
    d) are found in the environment

165) *Which ONE of the following systems is NOT an autoclave?*

a) Vertical pressure cooker
b) Horizontal or vertical downward
c) Horizontal pressure cooker
d) Vacuum assisted

166) *Which ONE of the following is NOT an autoclave temperature, pressure, time combination?*

a) 121°C 15psi 15 min
b) 123°C 17psi 13 min
c) 126°C 20psi 10 min
d) 134°C 30psi 3.5 min

167) *Which ONE of the following is the MINIMUM temperature recommended for a hot air oven?*

a) 130°C
b) 150°C
c) 160°C
d) 180°C

168) *Which ONE of the following should NOT be sterilized in a hot air oven?*

a) Glassware
b) Sharp cutting instruments
c) Swabs
d) Powders

169) *How should packs be placed in a vacuum assisted oven?*

   a) Horizontally
   b) Unwrapped
   c) Tightly packed
   d) Vertically

170) *Which ONE of the following is NOT part of an instrument cleaning routine?*

   a) Wash in cold water
   b) Wash in hot water
   c) Lubrication
   d) Rinsing

171) *Assuming no complications, how long after surgery should skin sutures be removed?*

   a) 2–3 days
   b) 4–5 days
   c) 7–10 days
   d) 15–17 days

172) *Which ONE of the following needle holders have scissors as well?*

   a) Mcphail
   b) Mayo–Hegar
   c) Debakey
   d) Olsen–Hagar

173) *Which ONE of the following retractors is NOT self-retaining?*

   a) Gossett
   b) Gelpi
   c) West
   d) Langenbeck

174) *Which ONE of the following types of retractors are self-retaining?*

   a) Gelpi
   b) Hohmann
   c) Langenbeck
   d) Volkmann

175) *A hot air oven sterilizes surgical instruments at:*

   a) 121°C
   b) 126°C
   c) 135°C
   d) Over 150°C

176) *Ethylene oxide is MOST commonly used to sterilize articles that:*

   a) are made of PVC
   b) cannot be dried effectively
   c) need to be sterilized quickly
   d) tend to be damaged by heat

177) *In what surgical procedure would you be MOST likely to use a periosteal elevator?*

a) Abdominal
b) Diaphragmatic
c) Ophthalmic
d) Orthopaedic

178) *A vertical pressure cooker works at:*

a) 15 psi at 121°C
b) 20psi at 128°C
c) 34 psi at 134°C
d) none of the above

179) *Which ONE of the following statements regarding hot air ovens is NOT true?*

a) They are economical
b) They do not corrode instruments
c) They have short sterilizing times
d) They are good for sterilizing glassware

180) *Which ONE of the following would NOT be sterilized by a hot air oven?*

a) Drill bits
b) Test tubes
c) Drapes
d) Liquids

181) *The environmental temperature in theatre should be maintained at:*

   a) 15°C
   b) 20°C
   c) 25°C
   d) 30°C

182) *Which ONE of the following scissors should be used for suture removal?*

   a) Metzebaum
   b) Mayo
   c) Lister
   d) Spencer

183) *In relation to suture material the word memory describes:*

   a) the ability of the suture material to undergo sterilization without deteriorating
   b) the lack of smoothness as the knot is tightened
   c) the tendency of the material to straighten out after loops have developed
   d) the response of the tissue to the suture material

184) *Which ONE of the following suture materials CANNNOT be autoclaved?*

   a) Polypropylene
   b) Polyester
   c) Nylon
   d) Polyglycolic Acid

185) *Polyglactin 910 is:*

    a) Vicryl
    b) Nylon
    c) PDS
    d) Dexon

186) *Which ONE of the following is an absorbable suture material?*

    a) Nylon
    b) Polypropylene
    c) Polyester
    d) Polyglycolic acid

187) *Which ONE of the following is NOT an essential precaution when using liquid nitrogen as a refrigerant in cryosurgery?*

    a) To make sure the stopper is always firmly screwed down on the container when not in use
    b) To ensure the room is well ventilated
    c) To use protective eye goggles
    d) To wear well-insulated gloves to avoid splashing liquid nitrogen on the hands

188) *Which ONE of the following suture materials is NOT absorbable?*

    a) Catgut
    b) Polydioxanone
    c) Polyglactin 910
    d) Polypropylene

189) *Which ONE of the following types of forceps is a bowel clamp?*

   a) Adson's
   b) Cheatle
   c) Doyen
   d) Gillies

190) *Which ONE of the following will NOT reduce the effectiveness of autoclaving in sterilizing surgical packs?*

   a) Dried blood left on instruments
   b) Overloading the autoclave
   c) Stacking packs without space between them
   d) Underfilling the autoclave

191) *Which ONE of the following scalpel blades requires a size 4 scalpel handle?*

   a) 10
   b) 11
   c) 15
   d) 20

192) *Why do some surgical instruments have gold- coloured handles?*

   a) To prevent rusting
   b) To prevent them becoming magnetized
   c) To reduce the build-up of static electricity
   d) To show they have tungsten inserts

193) *Why do some swabs have a black line in them?*

   a) To indicate their weight and absorbency
   b) To indicate they are not suitable for use in body cavities
   c) To make them easier to see when saturated with blood
   d) To make them visible on x-ray

194) *The DISADVANTAGE of using spore strips to check for effective sterilization is that:*

   a) they only check for spores, not viruses or bacteria
   b) they only indicate the temperature reached, not how long it was maintained
   c) they only work in an autoclave
   d) they require incubation after exposure, so the results are not known for several days

195) *The surgical gown should be folded before sterilization so that WHICH part of the gown is uppermost when the pack is opened?*

   a) The cuffs of the gown sleeve
   b) The inside of the gown shoulder seams
   c) The inside of the gown waist seam
   d) The outside of the gown waist

196) *What is a Volkmann's spoon?*

a) A curette
b) A lobe in the cerebellum of the brain
c) An indentation of the pelvis
d) An instrument used to dispense powders or granules

197) *What is the function of Spencer-Wells forceps?*

a) Haemostasis
b) Muscle retraction
c) Needle holding
d) Tissue holding

198) *What is the name of the needle holder used in ophthalmic surgical procedures?*

a) Castroviejo's
b) Debakey's
c) Kilner's
d) Mayo–Hagar's

199) *When draping a prepared surgical site (e.g. an abdomen for laparotomy), the first drape to be positioned should be the one:*

a) between the surgeon and the patient
b) nearest the head of the patient
c) nearest the tail of the patient
d) furthest from the surgeon

200) *When using a Browne's tube, what colour indicates*
that the correct temperature has been maintained for
the correct time?

a) Blue
b) Brown
c) Green
d) Orange

201) *Chromic catgut has been treated with chromium salts*
in order to:

a) increase its shelf life
b) make it less irritant to tissues
c) make it less likely to break down when knots are
tied
d) slow down the rate of breakdown within the body

202) *What type of needle SHOULD be used on delicate soft*
tissue?

a) a curved cutting needle
b) a round-bodied needle
c) a straight cutting needle
d) a taper-cut needle

203) *Glove powder is made from:*

a) antibiotic powder
b) maize starch
c) sodium bicarbonate
d) talcum powder

204) *When putting on surgical gloves before major surgery,*
which ONE of the following methods is recommended?

a) Closed gloving
b) Open gloving
c) Over-gloving
d) Plunge gloving

205) *Where should the earth plate of a diathermy machine*
be placed when in use?

a) Between the patient and the drapes
b) Between the patient and the rubber tabletop
c) Between the rubber tabletop and the table
d) On the floor beneath the table

206) *Which ONE of the following procedures should NOT*
be included in the daily cleaning routine in an operating
theatre?

a) All cleaning utensils should be used only in the
operating theatre, not in other parts of the
hospital
b) At the beginning of the day, wipe over all surfaces
with a dry cloth
c) At the end of the day, any loose hairs and debris
should be vacuumed up before washing the floor
d) Between operations, the operating table and any
soiled surfaces should be wiped clean

207) *Which ONE of the following skin preparations SHOULD be used prior to surgery round the eye and oral mucosa?*

   a) Chlorhexidine
   b) Povidine-iodine
   c) Surgical spirit
   d) Either a or b

208) *Surgical gloves are sterilized by which method?*

   a) Infra-red radiation
   b) Gamma radiation
   c) Ethylene oxide
   d) Autoclave

209) *Sterilization CANNOT be achieved by:*

   a) boiling
   b) hot air
   c) ethylene oxide
   d) autoclaving

210) *What is the potentially harmful chemical contained in CIDEX?*

   a) Formalin
   b) Bleach
   c) Gluteraldehyde
   d) Ethylene oxide

211) *Which ONE of the following methods of sterilization is MOST appropriate for a flexible endoscope?*

    a) Cold chemical sterilization

    b) Hot air

    c) Autoclave

    d) Gamma radiation

212) *Which scissors SHOULD be used for deep tissue dissection surgery?*

    a) Mayo

    b) Metzenbaum

    c) Potts

    d) Lister

213) *What is a Doyen clamp used for?*

    a) Holding and clamping the bowel

    b) Clamping blood vessels

    c) Holding a fractured end of bone for plating

    d) Clamping the uterus during ovariohysterectomy

214) *In order to move about the theatre, how SHOULD scrubbed personnel pass each other?*

    a) Any way that is convenient

    b) Back to back

    c) Back to front

    d) Front to front

215) *The holding time or sterilization time for instruments in an autoclave operating at a pressure of 30 psi and a temperature of 134C is:*

    a) 3.5 min
    b) 10 min
    c) 15 min
    d) 30 min

216) *Which size suture material is one size thicker than 3/0?*

    a) 2/0
    b) 4/0
    c) 1
    d) 0

217) *Which suture material is monofilament?*

    a) Silk
    b) Catgut
    c) Polypropylene
    d) Polyglactin 910

218) *Which one of the following suture materials is broken down by enzymes?*

    a) Polyglactin 910
    b) Polypropylene
    c) Polydioxanone
    d) Chromic catgut

219) *Why is it important NOT to get glove powder on the outside of surgical gloves?*

a) Not sterile
b) Causes haemorrhage
c) Irritant to tissues
d) Damages surgical instruments

220) *What type of suture needle SHOULD be used on delicate fibrous tissue?*

a) Taper-cut
b) Reverse cut
c) Curved cutting
d) Round-bodied

221) *Which ONE of the following suture materials is absorbable?*

a) Braided silk
b) Polyamide
c) Polyglactin 910
d) Polypropylene

222) *What does a Wright's respirometer do?*

a) Measures minute volume of the patient
b) Measures tidal volume of the patient
c) Measures respiration rate of the patient
d) Measures inspiration concentration of halothane

223) *A 30 kg dog is anaesthetized and maintained on a Magill circuit. What flow rate will be required if the dog is breathing about 20 times a minute?*

   a) 3–5 L/min
   b) 6–9 L/min
   c) 9–11 L/min
   d) 12–14 L/min

224) *A Lack circuit can be classified as which type of anaesthetic circuit?*

   a) Open
   b) Closed
   c) Semi-open
   d) Semi-closed

225) *Calculate the flow rates required of oxygen and nitrous oxide for a 15 kg dog to be maintained on a Lack circuit (assuming a minute volume of 200 ml/kg):*

   a) 1 L oxygen, 2 L nitrous oxide
   b) 1.5 L oxygen, 3.5 L nitrous oxide
   c) 2.5 L oxygen, 5 L nitrous oxide
   d) 3.5 L oxygen, 6.5 L nitrous oxide

226) *Calculate the volume of Saffan (12 mg/ml) required to anaesthetize a cat weighing 6 kg. The dose rate is 3 mg/kg:*

   a) 1ml
   b) 1.5ml
   c) 2ml
   d) 2.5ml

227) *Calculate the volume of 1.25% thiopentone required to anaesthetize a 3.75 kg dog. The dose rate is 10 mg/kg:*

   a) 2 ml
   b) 3 ml
   c) 4 ml
   d) 5 ml

228) *How much anaesthetic agent is there in 100 ml of a 5% solution?*

   a) 5 mg
   b) 50 mg
   c) 500 mg
   d) 5000 mg

229) *Identify the following circuit:*

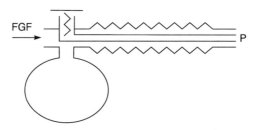

a) Ayres T-piece (Jackson-Rees modification)
b) Modified Bain
c) Lack
d) Magill

230) *Identify the following circuit:*

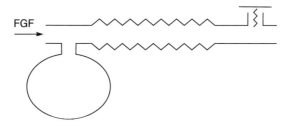

a) Ayres T-piece (Jackson-Rees modification)
b) Bain
c) Lack
d) Magill

231)   *Identify the following circuit:*

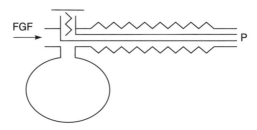

a) Ayres T-piece (Jackson-Rees modification)
b) Bain
c) Lack
d) Magill

232)   *Nitrous oxide comes in cylinders that are:*

a) black with white shoulders
b) blue
c) grey
d) orange

233)   *Oxygen is supplied in cylinders that are:*

a) Black with white shoulders
b) Blue
c) Grey
d) Orange

234) *The statement that a drug has a very high therapeutic index means:*

a) it is very easy to overdose using this drug
b) this drug can be given at several times its recommended dose rate with relative safety
c) this drug is very effective at its recommended dose rate
d) this drug may cause excitement on injection

235) *Which ONE of the following drugs is a benzodiazepine?*

a) Acepromazine
b) Buprenorphine
c) Diazepam
d) Ketamine

236) *Which ONE of the following is a dissociative anaesthetic?*

a) acepromazine
b) buprenorphine
c) diazepam
d) ketamine

237) *Which ONE of the following is NOT a controlled drug?*

a) Buprenorphine
b) Morphine
c) Pentobarbitone
d) Propofol

238) *Which ONE of the following is NOT a property of acepromazine?*

a) It is anti-emetic
b) It is contraindicated in dyspnoeic patients
c) It is contraindicated in epileptic patients
d) It is hypertensive

239) *Which ONE of the following is a property of nitrous oxide?*

a) It causes significant respiratory depression
b) It does not require scavenging
c) It is an analgesic
d) It is explosive

240) *Which ONE of the following is a schedule 2 controlled drug?*

a) Buprenorphine
b) Morphine
c) Pentobarbitone
d) Phenobarbitone

241) *Which ONE of the following is a schedule 3 controlled drug?*

a) Buprenorphine
b) Diazepam
c) Etorhine
d) Pethidine

242) *Which ONE of the following statements about ketamine is NOT true?*

    a) Ketamine produces minimal cardiovascular and respiratory depression

    b) Ketamine gives good analgesia

    c) Ketamine gives good muscle relaxation

    d) Ketamine tends to preserve the cough reflex

243) *Which ONE of the following statements about methohexitone is NOT true?*

    a) Animals make a much faster recovery from methohexitone than from thiopentone

    b) It is much faster acting than thiopentone

    c) It is twice/three times as potent as thiopentone

    d) Perivascular injection does not cause tissue damage as does thiopentone

244) *Which ONE of the following statements about propofol is NOT true?*

    a) It causes less respiratory depression that thiopentone

    b) It is non-cumulative when administered by infusion in dogs

    c) It often causes a transient apnoea on induction

    d) It should not be stored once the vial has been opened

245) *Which ONE of the following drugs is NOT classified as a barbiturate?*

   a) Thiopentone sodium
   b) Intraval
   c) Methohexitone
   d) Xylazine

246) *Which ONE of the following drugs is an opioid antagonist?*

   a) Naloxone
   b) Atropine
   c) Pancuronium
   d) Tolazine

247) *Which ONE of the following drugs is the antagonist of medetomidine?*

   a) Naloxone
   b) Flumazenil
   c) Tolazine
   d) Atipamazole

248) *Use of nitrous oxide in anaesthesia:*

   a) increases the amount of inhalational agent required
   b) decreases the amount of inhalational agent required
   c) slows the induction process
   d) has no effect on the time or amount of anaesthetic required

249) *Which ONE of the following is NOT a good reason to use a premedication?*

a) To calm the patient
b) To minimize the dose of induction agent required
c) To smooth induction and recovery
d) To increase vagal activity

250) *Which ONE of the following is NOT an advantage of endotracheal intubation?*

a) It ensures a patent airway
b) It increases the dead space
c) It prevents aspiration pneumonia
d) It allows us to carry out IPPV

251) *The oxygen flush valve on an anaesthetic machine:*

a) allows oxygen to flow into the breathing system without going through a vaporiser
b) increases the anaesthetic concentration within the circuit
c) causes the patient to breathe more deeply
d) is used primarily to keep the reservoir bag inflated

252) *The ADVANTAGES of a non rebreathing system, as
      compared with a rebreathing system, include all of the
      following EXCEPT:*

      a) reduced resistance to breathing
      b) greater potential for hypothermia caused by high
         flows needed
      c) reduced mechanical dead space
      d) no soda lime required

253) *Which ONE of the following has good analgesic
      properties?*

      a) Methohexitone sodium
      b) Propofol
      c) Isoflurane
      d) Nitrous oxide

254) *Which ONE of the following drugs is a depolarizing
      muscle relaxant?*

      a) Pancuronium
      b) Suxamethonium
      c) Atracurium
      d) Gallamine

255) *Cardiopulmonary arrest may be indicated by:*

      a) bright red bleeding at the surgical site
      b) constriction of the pupils
      c) respiratory arrest or gasping
      d) generalized muscle tension

256) *Which ONE of the following anaesthetic circuits MIGHT lead to hyperthermia in an anaesthetized patient?*

   a) Ayres T-piece
   b) To and fro
   c) Magill
   d) Circle

257) *If a 10 kg dog has a tidal volume of 15 ml/kg and a respiratory rate of 20 breaths/minute, what flow rate would you use if it was connected to a Bains circuit?*

   a) 4–6 L/min
   b) 7.5–9 L/min
   c) 10–12 L/min
   d) 15–18 L/min

258) *How many mg/ml are there in a 4% solution?*

   a) 0.4 mg
   b) 4 mg
   c) 40 mg
   d) 400 mg

259) *What is a Water's canister and what is the function of this piece of equipment?*

 a) A device on an anaesthetic machine which allows humidification of the gases

 b) An old and inaccurate type of vaporiser

 c) A canister containing soda lime which is part of a to and fro circuit

 d) Part of a rebreathing circuit which absorbs nitrous oxide

260) *Calculate the flow rates of oxygen and nitrous oxide for a 30 kg dog to be maintained on a Magill circuit (assuming a minute volume of 200 ml/kg):*

 a) 1.25 L oxygen, 2.5 L nitrous oxide

 b) 1.75 L oxygen, 3.25 L nitrous oxide

 c) 2.0 L oxygen, 4.0 L nitrous oxide

 d) 2.75 L oxygen, 6.5 L nitrous oxide

261) *Identify the following circuit:*

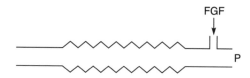

 a) Ayres T-piece

 b) Bain

 c) Lack

 d) Magill

262) *When monitoring the vital signs of an anaesthetized patient, which one of the following must you record?*

a) Mucous membrane colour and capillary refill time
b) Heart rate and respiratory rate and depth
c) Jaw and eye reflexes
d) All of the above

263) *Using ketamine as an anaesthetic agent diminishes the value of which measure in assessing anaesthetic depth?*

a) Pedal reflex
b) Jaw muscle tone
c) Eye position
d) Anal reflex

264) *Adrenaline is included in local anaesthetic preparations for the following reason:*

a) it aids the absorption of the lignocaine into the CNS
b) it aids the rapid dispersal of the drug throughout the body
c) it causes local vasoconstriction, keeping the drug where it is placed for a longer period of time
d) it reduces the likelihood of a decrease in heart rate due to the effect of the lignocaine

265) *An ataractic drug produces:*

  a) a calming effect
  b) a decrease in saliva production
  c) an increase in excitability
  d) an increase in heart rate

266) *Atropine is:*

  a) a non-steroidal anti-inflammatory
  b) a tranquillizer
  c) an antipyretic
  d) an antisialogogue

267) *Open, part-used vials of Propofol should be disposed of:*

  a) after 48 hours at room temperature
  b) after 24 hours in a refrigerator
  c) after 7 days in a refrigerator
  d) at the end of each day

268) *The occasional anaphylactic reactions seen in cats following injection of Saffan are due to:*

  a) anaesthetic overdose
  b) perivascular injection of the anaesthetic
  c) reaction to the alphaxolone
  d) reaction to the Cremophor EL

269) *A cat requires sedation with a 2% solution of xylazine. The dose rate is 3mg/kg. The cat weighs 4 kg. How many ml of the solution are required?*

   a) 0.6 ml
   b) 0.3 ml
   c) 6 ml
   d) 0.06 ml

270) *How much anaesthetic agent is there in 100 ml of 2.5% solution?*

   a) 2.5 g
   b) 25 mg
   c) 250 mg
   d) 250 g

271) *The dose rate for buprenorphine is 0.006 mg/kg. The concentration of the solution is 0.3 mg/ml. How many ml does a 5 50 kg Rottweiler require?*

   a) 0.1 ml
   b) 0.5 ml
   c) 1 ml
   d) 2 ml

272) *How much (in ml) of thiopentone should be drawn up ready to anaesthetize a premedicated dog weighing 20 kg? The dose rate is 10 mg /kg and the solution is 2.5%:*

a) 8 ml
b) 10 ml
c) 20 ml
d) 6 ml

273) *How many milligrams are required to make up 100 ml of a 5% solution of thiopentone?*

a) 5000 mg
b) 5 mg
c) 50 mg
d) 0.5 mg

274) *What is the total flow rate for a 30 kg Labrador with a respiratory rate of 15 breaths per minute on a Lack circuit?*

a) 4.5–6.75 L/min
b) 6.75–8 L/min
c) 8–12.75 L/min
d) 10–12.5 L/min

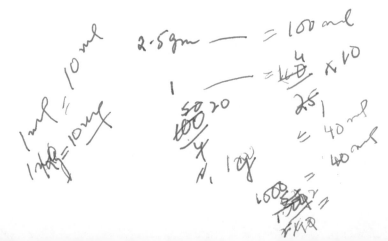

275) *What is the minute volume of a 5 kg cat breathing 20 times a minute?*

a) 100 ml/min
b) 1500 ml/min
c) 150 ml/min
d) 1000 ml/min

276) *The tidal volume is described as:*

a) the total lung capacity
b) the residual capacity
c) the amount of air inspired and expired in one breath
d) the amount of air inspired only

277) *What is the estimated tidal volume of a 20 kg dog?*

a) 4000 ml
b) 2000 ml
c) 1000 ml
d) 3000 ml

278) *Which ONE of the following is a rebreathing circuit?*

a) Bains
b) Ayres T-piece
c) Circle
d) Lack

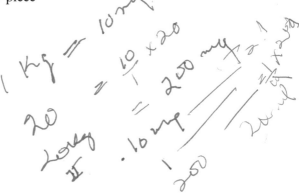

279) *Which ONE of the following is NOT a peripheral artery?*

   a) Femoral
   b) Tarsal
   c) Sub-lingual
   d) Coccygeal

280) *What is the portion of tidal volume called, where no gaseous exchange takes place?*

   a) Reservoir
   b) Minute volume
   c) Dead space
   d) Circuit volume

281) *What does hypercapnia mean?*

   a) Excess of carbon dioxide
   b) Lack of carbon dioxide
   c) Excess of nitrous oxide
   d) Lack of nitrous oxide

282) *All of the following anaesthetics can be used in the dog EXCEPT:*

   a) ketamine
   b) propofol
   c) alphaxalone/alphadolone
   d) methohexitone sodium

283) *Which ONE of the following anaesthetic drugs would be MOST suitable for anaesthetizing a greyhound?*

   a) Propofol
   b) Thiopentone
   c) Sagatal
   d) Halothane

284) *Which ONE of the following is FALSE?*

   a) Propofol is non-cumulative when administered by infusion in dogs
   b) Propofol should not be stored when the vial is opened
   c) Propofol may cause a transient apnoea following induction
   d) Propofol is less of a respiratory depressant than thiopentone

285) *The premedicant agent which has significant analgesic effects is:*

   a) acepromazine
   b) buprenorphine
   c) atropine
   d) diazepam

286) *Which ONE of the following is NOT an opioid?*

   a) Pethidine
   b) Morphine
   c) Papaveretum
   d) Flunixin

287) *The agent that can be used to reverse the effects of Small Animal Immobilon in man is:*

a) naloxone
b) neostigmine
c) atipamazole
d) etorphine

288) *Anticholinergics are often included in premedication for cats and dogs:*

a) to produce pupil dilatation
b) to decrease saliva and bronchial secretions
c) to decrease the amount of induction agent required
d) to calm the animal

289) *Which opioid agent may require IPPV if given during surgery for analgesia?*

a) Morphine
b) Pethidine
c) Buprenorphine
d) Fentanyl

290) *Which ONE of the following has the LOWEST MAC value?*

a) Methoxyflurane
b) Halothane
c) Nitrous oxide
d) Isoflurane

291) *The anaesthetic gas supplied in blue cylinders is:*

a) oxygen
b) nitrous oxide
c) carbon dioxide
d) cyclopropane

292) *What does MAC stand for?*

a) Maximum alveolar concentration
b) Minimum alveolar concentration
c) Minimum anaesthetic concentration
d) Minimum alveolar coefficient

293) *To be considered effective, nitrous oxide SHOULD be used in concentrations of:*

a) 20%
b) 40%
c) 70%
d) none of the above

294) *Recovery from methohexitone compared to thiopentone will be:*

a) faster
b) same
c) slower
d) dependent on the breed of animal

295) *Which ONE of the following is NOT a valid reason for administering a premedication?*

a) To reduce the total amount of general anaesthetic required for induction
b) To calm an excited animal
c) To increase patient safety by allowing the animal to stay under general anaesthetic longer
d) To reduce pain in the postoperative period

296) *The pop-off valve on an anaesthetic machine helps to:*

a) vaporise the liquid anaesthetic
b) prevent excess gas building up within the circuit
c) prevent waste gas re-entering the vaporiser
d) keep the oxygen flowing in one direction

297) *An obese dog about to receive an injectable anaesthetic should receive:*

a) the dose prescribed on a mg/kg basis
b) a reduced dosage
c) a dosage based on ideal weight
d) an inhalation anaesthetic only

298) *Which ONE of the following drugs, often used as premedicants, is sometimes contraindicated for use in Boxers?*

a) Glycopyrrolate
b) Acepromazine
c) Diazepam
d) Atropine

299) *As the animal becomes anaesthetized, which one of the following is the first reflex to be lost?*

   a) Pedal
   b) Anal
   c) Swallowing
   d) Palpebral

300) *Which ONE of the following pH values is closest to the pH of thiopentone sodium?*

   a) 2.4
   b) 6.4
   c) 8.4
   d) 10.4

Answers

1)	c	23)	b	45)	c	67)	d
2)	c	24)	b	46)	a	68)	c
3)	a	25)	d	47)	d	69)	b
4)	a	26)	c	48)	b	70)	b
5)	c	27)	a	49)	c	71)	b
6)	c	28)	c	50)	b	72)	d
7)	b	29)	a	51)	d	73)	a
8)	d	30)	b	52)	c	74)	a
9)	b	31)	c	53)	a	75)	a
10)	d	32)	d	54)	c	76)	c
11)	a	33)	b	55)	d	77)	a
12)	d	34)	d	56)	b	78)	c
13)	d	35)	c	57)	c	79)	a
14)	b	36)	b	58)	b	80)	b
15)	c	37)	c	59)	b	81)	a
16)	c	38)	b	60)	b	82)	a
17)	b	39)	a	61)	d	83)	d
18)	a	40)	c	62)	c	84)	a
19)	d	41)	a	63)	b	85)	d
20)	b	42)	d	64)	c	86)	b
21)	b	43)	b	65)	a	87)	d
22)	b	44)	b	66)	b	88)	b

89)	d	125)	c	161)	d	197)	a
90)	b	126)	c	162)	c	198)	a
91)	c	127)	d	163)	c	199)	a
92)	c	128)	b	164)	b	200)	c
93)	d	129)	b	165)	c	201)	b
94)	b	130)	d	166)	b	202)	b
95)	d	131)	a	167)	b	203)	b
96)	c	132)	d	168)	c	204)	a
97)	b	133)	b	169)	d	205)	b
98)	c	134)	b	170)	b	206)	b
99)	c	135)	c	171)	c	207)	b
100)	b	136)	b	172)	d	208)	b
101)	c	137)	d	173)	d	209)	a
102)	a	138)	a	174)	a	210)	c
103)	b	139)	a	175)	d	211)	a
104)	b	140)	b	176)	d	212)	b
105)	c	141)	c	177)	d	213)	a
106)	d	142)	b	178)	a	214)	b
107)	b	143)	c	179)	c	215)	a
108)	c	144)	c	180)	c	216)	a
109)	a	145)	b	181)	b	217)	c
110)	b	146)	b	182)	d	218)	d
111)	b	147)	a	183)	c	219)	c
112)	d	148)	c	184)	d	220)	a
113)	d	149)	c	185)	a	221)	c
114)	c	150)	b	186)	d	222)	b
115)	d	151)	b	187)	b	223)	b
116)	b	152)	d	188)	d	224)	d
117)	d	153)	b	189)	c	225)	a
118)	d	154)	a	190)	d	226)	b
119)	d	155)	d	191)	d	227)	b
120)	c	156)	b	192)	d	228)	d
121)	c	157)	c	193)	d	229)	c
122)	b	158)	b	194)	d	230)	d
123)	a	159)	b	195)	b	231)	c
124)	a	160)	a	196)	a	232)	b

233)	a	250)	b	267)	d	284)	d
234)	b	251)	a	268)	d	285)	b
235)	c	252)	b	269)	a	286)	d
236)	d	253)	d	270)	a	287)	a
237)	d	254)	b	271)	c	288)	b
238)	d	255)	c	272)	a	289)	d
239)	c	256)	b	273)	a	290)	a
240)	b	257)	b	274)	a	291)	b
241)	a	258)	c	275)	b	292)	b
242)	c	259)	c	276)	c	293)	c
243)	d	260)	b	277)	a	294)	a
244)	a	261)	a	278)	c	295)	c
245)	d	262)	d	279)	a	296)	b
246)	a	263)	c	280)	c	297)	c
247)	d	264)	c	281)	a	298)	b
248)	b	265)	a	282)	c	299)	c
249)	d	266)	d	283)	a	300)	d